How I increase my height without any oral medicine.

"Working steps of height increasing after puberty without any oral medicine."

Mahesh Kaushik

www.popati.blogspot.com

Preface

You purchased this book because you want to grow taller; your hard earned money not going to waste if you are ready to follow this unique height increase program. 1-3 inches of height gain is possible if you practice it with faith and patience. People below 18 years of age get better results(near about 3-7 inch). But after puberty, it will be 0.1 to 3 inches only. Overall results depending on your faith, age, body, diet, and practice.

I have described this height increase program in my blog http://popati.blogspot.com/ since last 4 years.

Popati height increase program is the world famous four step height increase program.
1. Step: - Doing meditation.
2. Step: - Change food habits.
3. Step: - Acupressure.
4. Step: - One simple exercise.

This book is not just a copy paste of my blog articles. This book is written to describe complete point to point system of height increase and it will be sure give you benefit and *of course you no need to oral medication, no need for steroidal growth formulas and no need to hard exercises.*

This book cannot give you any about any certain level of height increase but I think if you follow all the ideas you will be gaining some mm to inches in your height. Please remember the result may be differing from person to person.

Mahesh Chander Kaushik

Email me your progress and suggestions:- mahesh2073@yahoo.com

(I get 100 of emails per day from my Popati blog readers and followers of my stock market blog so it is impossible for me to reply every mail but I try to reply to most of my mails. If you ask any query that really needs a reply, then I would be happy to reply you, please do not mail me spam because my spam detection software automatic delete all mails containing links and spam's).

-: Table of contents:-

1
How I invented this height increase technique.

I am a spiritual person and at the age of 35 years I start inner meditation for getting spiritual power. This inner meditation also known as Agya chakra meditation (also known as ajna chakra meditation or eyebrow center meditation) or inner tratka in Hinduism.

Actually I read a book about meditation for spiritual power and follow the tratka meditation for getting spiritual power , it is a different subject that I get spiritual power or not but after practice of 2-3 months I noticed that my height is increasing. I think I got one inch at the age of 35 years .

Because my pants are short and my wife and friends tell me "that I look longer." It was a miracle for me so I am so exited and put all of my concentration on height increase instead of getting spiritual powers, finally it will increase near 3 inches.

I have never mapped my height so I can not provide an exact idea that how many inches I get added on to my height but since my puberty my elder brother is 3 inches taller than me but after this meditation and acupressure in the age of 35 I wonder that I reach my elder brother's height. So I think I gained 3 inches in my height.

Now I start research regarding why it happens? And I have developed a complete program to increase height without any oral medication. I called this program "Popati: Height increase program" (as you knew Popati is the name of my blog for alternative methods of healing).

2
What is Popati: Height increase program?

This program is the world's simplest and a cost free program of height increase to increase your height without spending any cost or fees of this program.

I divided it into four parts:-

1. **Meditation: -** It wants your 5 to 10 minutes per day but you will do it without spending any money.
2. **Food:** - Just add some low cost vegetarian foods in your daily diet for optimized results.
3. **Acupressure:** - It wants your 5 to 10 minutes per day but you will do it without spending any money.
4. **Only one exercise:** - It wants your 5 to 10 minutes per day but you will do it without spending any money

So this height increase program wants your practice faith and 15-30 minutes of your life. I knew you had no time but height is gift of god so 15-30 minutes is not a very high cost for this god gift.

So in the next article I told you that how anyone height is increased after puberty?

3
How Agya chakra or eyebrow center meditations increase height after puberty?

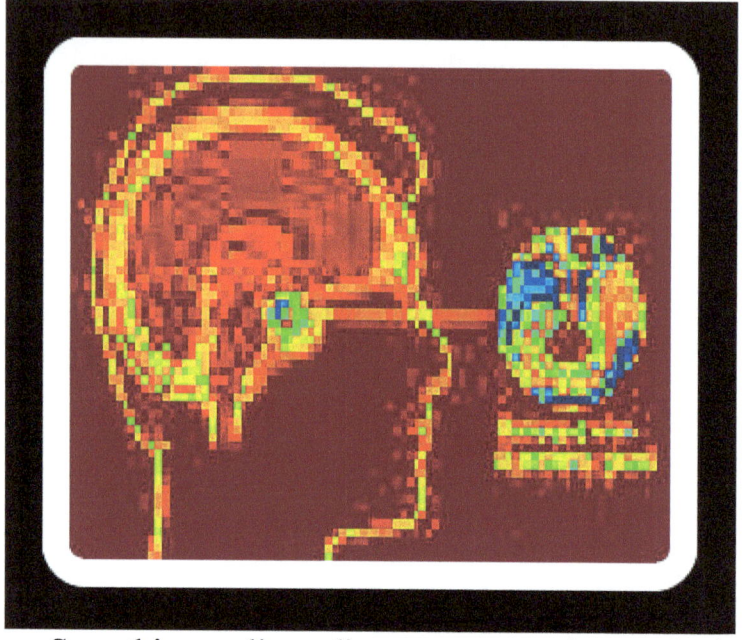

-: See this outline diagram to understand the location of pituitary gland in your forehead:-

First of all we try to learn the science behind height increase. Human growth hormone "Somatotropin" is responsible for height increase. This growth hormone is secreted by the pituitary gland so our height depended on our pituitary gland hormone.

The Agya Chakra is situated in the middle of the forehead (between the eyebrows) and Pituitary gland is located in the center of the skull, just behind the bridge of the nose (I think ancient yogic term Agya Chakra and modern medical science term Pituitary gland are same).

Our pituitary gland is about the size of a pea. It is the point which called Agya chakra or Anjna chakra in the language of meditation.

This method is working any age group because in yoga this meditation technique is called Agya Chkra meditation or inner tratka. This will give Anima or Laghima Sidhi.

(Anima Sidhi means: - A spiritual power that able the person to decrease size of their physical body , Laghima Sidhi means: - A spiritual power that able the person to reduce weight of their physical body)

You know that our monks have these sidhis Anima or laghima, which will be completely control of pituitary gland hormone, so if you try to simple meditation or follow other method, you will easily increase your height instead of sidhis (spiritual powers).

When we try to concentrate on this point our pituitary gland is stimulated or when we take a simple 5-20 minute meditation on the pituitary gland and think this part is stimulated and work more effectively. (In the next article of this book I give you more details that how you done it.)

We see magic effect of this meditation after 2-3 months.

Thousands of my followers find very good results.
Read this link and all of comments in this article where my followers report that they get results from this height increase meditation
http://popati.blogspot.in/2009/03/how-to-increase-your-height-no-pills-no.html

4
How to do height increase meditation?

It is so simple to start this meditation and grow near about 3 inches taller at any age.

Just draw this diagram on a white paper and fill the colors as shown in the diagram outer border have cream color, main circle has black color and inner circle have a yellow color.

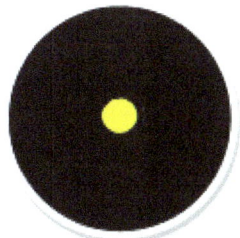

-: Picture for height increase meditation:-

Now fix this paper on a wall and sit down in front of this magic circle.

Please remember the level of your eyes and level of yellow circle is must be same as shown in next picture.

Now just concentrate your mind on the inner yellow circle and think " rays of this yellow circle interact with my pituitary gland and stimulate them for increasing my height."

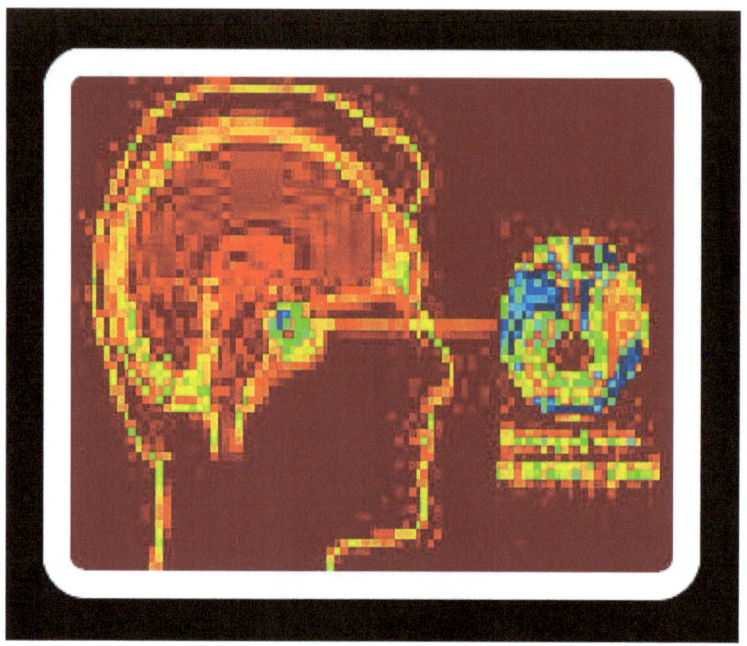

-:Picture:-outline of pituitary gland meditation and how this imagination of pituitary gland show in closed eyes:-

See the yellow circle without blinking your eyes until tears come when tears come close your eyes, now you see a reflection of this magic circle in the closed eyes just concentrate in this reflection and think again " My height is increasing" " my pituitary gland is stimulated and work more effectively."

Doing this meditation 2-10 minute per day it will be taken 30-60 days to get results.

One other meditation technique is described in my blog Popati read it on here :-
http: //popati. blogspot. in/2010/07/step-by-step-meditation-for-grow-height. html
Caution:-

1. If your eyesight is weak then do not force on eye take it easy , forcefully stopping of eye blinking is not recommended to just hold your eye blinking as you easily hold.
2. If you feel headache during the practice of meditation, then it is a sign that you doing it forcefully so stop it for some days and then restart again without force.
3. If the tear is not coming and you want to close your eye then no problem you just close the eye and start imagining of this black circle with yellow point in middle of your eyes.
4. All exercises and meditation is must be done under the care of expert teacher of yoga and meditation because the author is not liable for any harm.
5. Wash your eyes with normal cold water after meditation.

5
Food for height increase

Now you read the first part of this height increase program. Second part of this program is "Add some food item in your regular diet."

Two things are responsible for your height.The first thing bone size and second thing is the human growth hormone "Somatotropin".

Somatotropin hormone stimulates growth (height) by cell reproduction and regeneration.

Bone size depends on calcium intake.

Somatotropin is a protein base hormone so it depends on protein intake.

When you meditate for height increase, please take high calcium and high protein base diet. Take milk or high calcium foods because calcium is the main part of your bones and it helps increase your bone size.

So I think you may understand this simple science that "if you take food with a high density of protein and calcium will automatically increase your height due to increasing in bone size and stimulating human growth hormone secretion.

Suppose if you have done proper meditation or acupressure for height increase but not to eat protein based foods or calcium diet then it is impossible to create growth hormone somatotropin by the pituitary gland because human growth hormone is a peptide base hormone and protein foods is an essential requirement for secretion and creation of growth hormone.

So use lentils in your daily food specially "chickpea (Bengal gram)" have essentials amino acids for growth hormone. There are 2 types of chickpeas available in market first black use black chickpea for height increase benefit. Eat cheese containing foods because cheese also contains essential amino acids for height increase.

Avoid non vegetarian foods and eggs during this practice of height increase because I believe (not scientifically proven) that protein of non vegetarians foods and eggs increase level of Growth hormone-inhibiting hormone somatostatin that inhibits secretion of somatotropin. And in Hinduism this practice of meditation called Aghya Charka meditation which is a spiritual practice and avoiding of non vegetarian foods is a must requirement for stimulating the agya chakra (pituitary gland).

Lemon and citrus fruit may increase absorption of calcium and protein so add lemon and citrus fruits in your daily diet.

And excessive sugar or caffeine intake reduces the serum calcium level so try to avoiding them

So during the meditation period food that included your diet is

1. Chickpeas.
2. Lentils.
3. Beans.
4. Cheese
5. Milk
6. Lemmon and other citrus fruits.

And food that excluded in your diet includes:-

1. Eggs.
2. Non vegetarian products.
3. No excessive sugar or caffeine intake because they reduce the serum calcium level.

6
Acupressure for height increase

Third part of our height increase program is Acupressure.

When we give pressure on certain points of the body it will stimulate the nervous system that increases related hormone secretion so put pressure 5-15 minutes on your all thumbs upper front points (both hands and both legs thumb) see picture in this book where the acupressure points shown in red dots.

This acupressure also improves level of pituitary Hormon.

Red circles shown in these pictures are acupressure points for height increase.

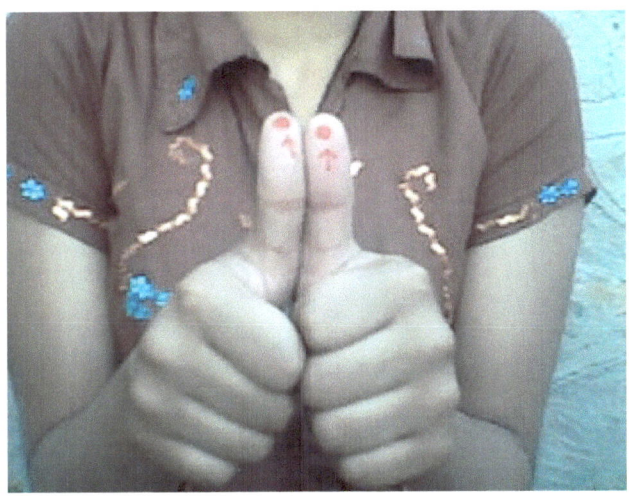

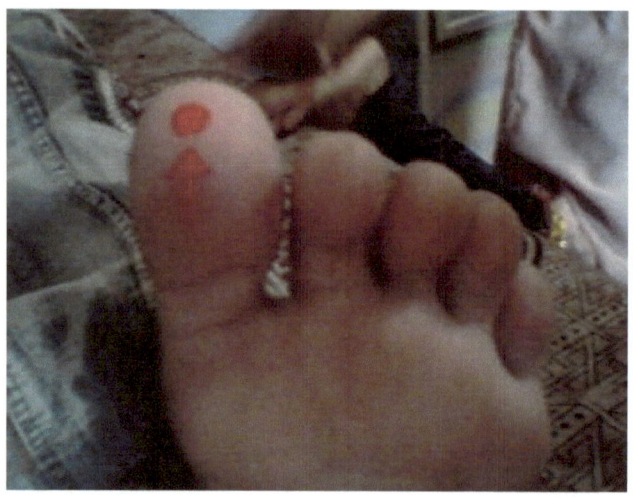

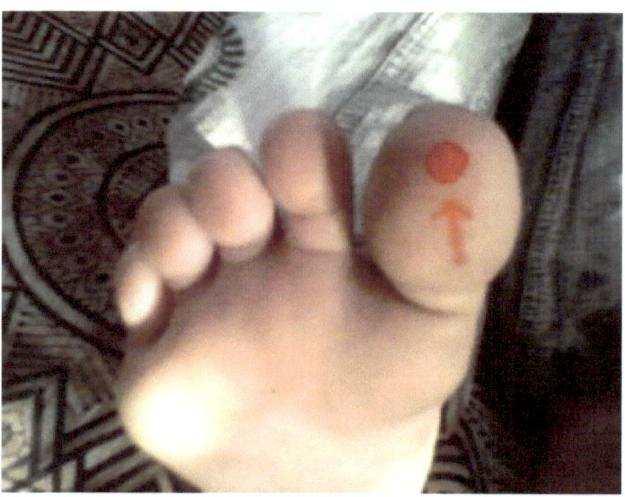

-: acupressure points for height increase are shown in red dots in the diagram:-

Pressure the points in 1-1-1-1-1-1 minute cycle, put pressure and then release repeatedly, press until you feel some uneasiness or feel little pain but minimum 1 minute is necessary to release growth hormone.

7
One stretch exercise for height increase

In the 11th century an Indian yogi named Shri Gorakshanath Ji invented a yogic exercise for height increase name Paschimottanasana.

This is a very powerful exercise so we included it in our height increase program. This is the fourth and last part of your height increase program

Warning: - please do Paschimottanasana under the care of your physiotherapist. You will have not to force with your spine because the author of this book is not liable for any harm of your spine during the practice of these asanas.

For doing Paschimottanasana

1. Sit up on the ground and straight with your legs together, stretch the legs stiff like a stick. Try catching the toes with the thumb, index and middle fingers. While catching, you will have to bend the trunk forwards.

2. Exhale and slowly bend spine until your forehead touches your knees. Do not force this; just try it slowly. After regular practice for 20-30 days, elasticity of your spine is up. You can keep the face between the knees also.

3. Be sure to during the **Paschimottanasana** keep the feet pointed straight up towards the ceiling and together.

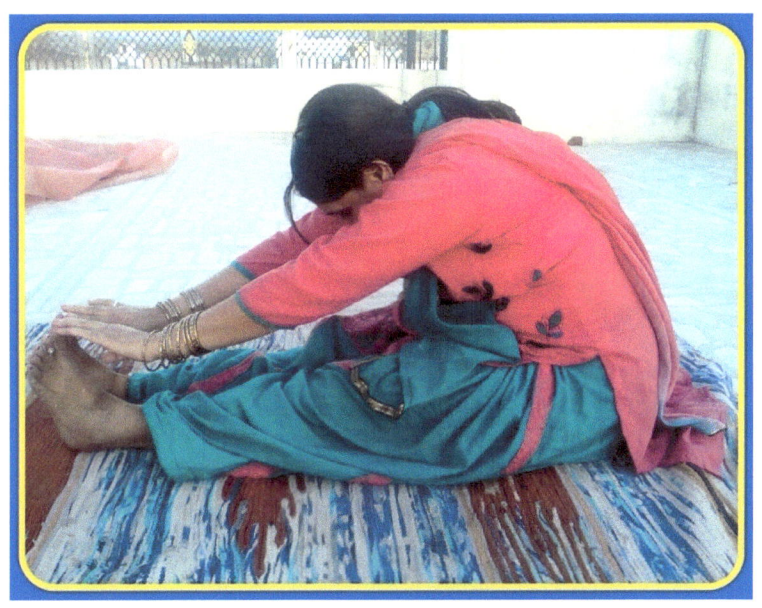

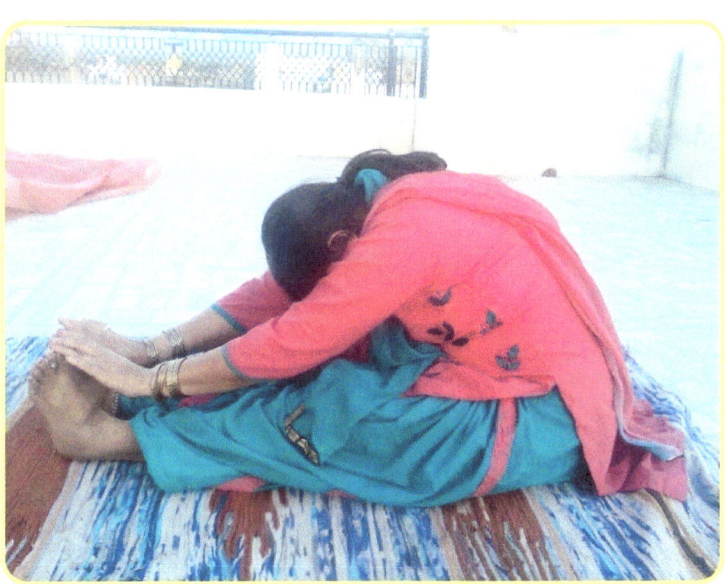

4. You will have not to force with your spine because the author of this book is not liable for any harm of your spine during the practice of these asanas.
5. So please do Paschimottanasana under the care of your physiotherapist.

For a deeper understanding of Paschimottanasana you will be see some video of Paschimottanasana on YouTube and search Paschimottanasana on google. In my meditation method 1 recommended practice of Paschimottanasana 5 minutes per day for optimized results.

8
How to map your height?

When you map your height by an inch-tape, then it will not be given to good result because if you stretch and loose the tape it will be 1-2 inch difference in stretch and loose mapping. So use only corner of wall method.

In this corner of the wall method, please stand at the corner of a room and ask someone to mark your height on corner wall with the help of marker pen. Do not use tape to mapping your height. Corner wall method is the right method of height marking.

After 21 days more of practice again mark it. If a difference is shown then you will continue your practice because it is free and you have nothing to lose.

9
Sex and height

There are a direct relation in sex and height during puberty. In puberty androgen secretion is increased (In males from testis and in females from adrenal cortex), This increased androgen secretion during puberty stimulate growth hormone (GH) secretion.

So if you control your sexual desire then your androgen level is increased and higher androgen levels stimulate growth hormone secretion.

But if you do sexual activity more frequently then your androgen level is reduced and it gives a negative effect on height increase.

So during the first 40 days of your height increase practice complete monastic celibacy (means no sex) is recommended for the best results, but if it is not possible then maintain minimum 7 days gap during the each intercourse for optimized results.

Control of sex is not a part of our height increase program but it is required for good results.

Side benefits of this program

When you take medicines, you got side effects but in this height increase practice you get some extra benefits such as:-

1. After some days of practice you see your eye sight is improving. Some of my followers claim that they get rid of their glasses as well as increasing their height.
2. You feel very calm and your anger stress and negative thinking are going away.
3. If you practice it you may get some spiritual power mostly you see coming events of your life in your dreams and wonder that events you see in your dreams is happening as it is in your life.
4. If you really done it spiritually and try to concentrate more than 20 minutes in closed eyes then some of followers claim that they see holy spiritual lightning yellow-green and sparkling light in their eyebrow center and if they pray a spiritual wish to this light then it is fulfill.

But please note author of this book not claim that you got all of these benefits because it all depend on your dedication, faith and practice.

I am not giving you any guarantee that this program is working, but I request you that please try it and if you really increases your height with the help of this free program then please make your true comments on my Popati blog , Facebook page and write reviews on Amazon or other book selling sites for help of others.

FAQ about height increase program

Question1. Can this method increase height at any age group?

Answer1: - this method will work for any age group because in yoga this meditation technique is called Agya Chakra dhayan or inner tratka this will give Anima or Laghima Sidhi.

You know that our monks have these sidhis Anima or laghima, which will be completely control of pituitary gland hormone, and if you try to simply meditate or follow other method, you will easily increase your height instead of sidhis.

But if you are below 24 then you find better results and below 20 years age people gain very much from this program.

Question 2: -Will this also increase height in people with fused growth plates. If so how is this possible since if your growth plates are closed it doesn't matter how much hormones you produce you can't grow?

Answer 2:- this method is spiritual (meditation) is a spiritual method not scientific method and in spirituality we not believe in growth plate fusion theory.So follow this method after the consult of your doctor and if your faith on meditation is allow you.

In hypnosis theory - Meditation or chakra opening for height increase is working at any age. The theory behind this is " if you can control your mind you can control your body."

Question 3: -_ I want to know that can we use something like a pencil for acupressure? Like the top of pencil for acupressure?
Answer 3: - Yes one can use pencil bottom for acupressure.

Question 4: - How much will I increase my height if I follow all of the points like meditation, acupressure, stretch exercises and foods?
Answer4 : - It depends on your body and age _so this book cannot guarantee you about any certain level of height increasing but I think 1-3 inch is possible if you practice it with faith and patience. People below 18 years of age get better results, near about 3-7 inch. But after puberty it will be 0.1 to 3 inches only depend on your faith and practice._

Question 5: - What is the best time for meditation?
Answer 5: - Early in the morning before sunrise is the best time for height increase meditation. The

second best time is just before sleep (bedtime) at night.

Question6: - what is the best time for acupressure?

Answer 6: - Any time of day.

Question 7: - what is the best time of stretch exercise?

Answer 7: - Early in the morning after bowel movement and empty stomach.

12
Summary of this book

Congrats! Now you read this book and ready to increase your height near 3 inches with the help of this program.

First of all please decide to follow all of the tips given in this book because only you knew that height is an important factor for you.

Okay, I am sure that if you follow tips give here then you will be getting results in 0.01 mm to 7 inches. It all depends on your age and practice of program.

Now ,read this summary again and start your try of height increase:-

1. Draw this diagram on a white paper and fill the colors as shown in the diagram outer border have cream color, main circle has black color and inner circle have a yellow color.

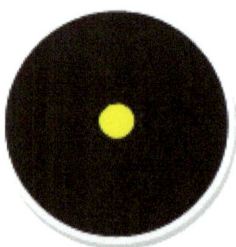

-: Picture for height increase meditation:-

Now fix this paper on a wall and sit down in front of this magic circle. See the yellow circle without blinking your eyes until tears come when tears come close your eye, now you see a reflection of this magic circle in closed eye just concentrate in this reflection and think again " My height is increasing" " my pituitary gland is stimulated and work more effectively" made it 5-15 minutes per day.

2. During this meditation period food that included your diet is

> Chickpeas.
> Lentils.
> Beans.
> Cheese.
> Milk.
> Lemmon and other citrus fruits.

Food that excluded in your diet includes Eggs.

> Non vegetarian products.
> No excessive sugar or caffeine intake because they reduce the serum calcium level.

3.Done acupressure for height increase for this purpose put pressure 5 -15 minutes on your all thumbs upper front points (both hands and both legs thumbs) as described earlier in this book.

4. Doing Paschimottanasana 5 minutes per day.
5. During the first 40 days of your height increase practice, complete monastic celibacy (means no sex) is recommended for best result but if it is not possible then maintain minimum 7 days gap during the each intercourse for optimized results.

If you really get benefited from this book then please make your true comments and positive review for help of others like you. You can also visit our Facebook page at this link

http://www.facebook.com/pages/Height-increase/136834929719630

Author book on stock market

If you enjoyed this book and find it is beneficial for you then you will be also like my book on stock market name **"The winning theory in stock market."** Read this exclusive book on the stock market at Amazon now.
http://www.amazon.com/dp/B00B2JM2BI

Author book on Laser hair removal

My exclusive book on laser hair removal also available online at Amazon read this at this link

http://www.amazon.com/Laser-parlour-guide-hair-removal/dp/1490369007